A Precious Bit of Forever

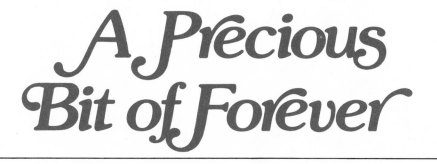

A Precious Bit of Forever

by Diane Head

Photographs by Evelyn R. Zeek
Design by David Koechel

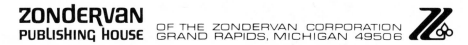

ZONDERVAN PUBLISHING HOUSE OF THE ZONDERVAN CORPORATION GRAND RAPIDS, MICHIGAN 49506

I would like to give special thanks to the people who helped make this book a reality . . .

CLYDE M. NARRAMORE and JEANETTE LOCKERBIE for believing in something yet unborn.

BRUCE and KATHY NARRAMORE for thoughts and inspiration stemming from the very first days of *Help! I'm a Parent.*

MARIHELEN WESTRICK and LINDA UDELL for loving words of gentle encouragement.

My mother, ELIZABETH HILL, and my mother-in-law, MILDRED HEAD, for loving hours spent with Melinda during the writing of this book.

A Precious Bit of Forever

"Buds of Promise" and "Dreams Do Come True" from *Poems for Mothers* by Phyllis C. Michael, © 1963 by Phyllis C. Michael. Used by permission.

"What Is a Girl?" and "What Is a Boy?" by Alan Beck, © 1950, used through the courtesy of New England Mutual Life Insurance Company.

"Birth," by Annie R. Stillman (Grace Raymond), from *The World's Best Poetry*, Vol. I: Of Home: Of Friendship, © 1904 by John D. Morris and Company, Philadelphia, Pa.

Scripture from *The Living Bible*, © 1971 by Tyndale House Publishers, Wheaton, Illinois. Used by permission.

A PRECIOUS BIT OF FOREVER
© 1976 by The Zondervan Corporation
Grand Rapids, Michigan

Second printing   March 1977

Library of Congress Cataloging in Publication Data
Head, Diane, 1945-
   A precious bit of forever.

   1. Pregnancy.   2. Childbirth.   3. Parent and
child.   I. Title.
RG525.H35   612.6   75-38722

Printed in the United States of America

To
Robert Lee
and our precious bit of forever,
Melinda Leigh

Contents

Buds
of
Promise

Just a bud
Of a blossom,
And yet —
What a promise
Of beauty
Full blown
And free!

Just a bit
Of a child,
But, oh,
What a vision
Of things
That are
To be!

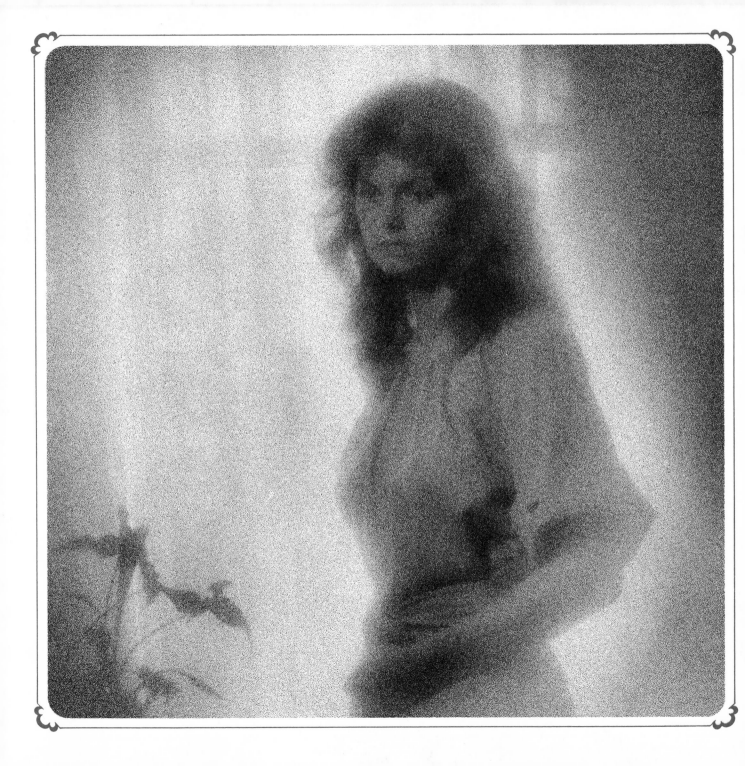

Part One

"For I am fearfully and wonderfully made."

— *Psalm 139:14* (KJV)

A Precious Bit of Forever

Suddenly the world has taken on a new glow! The robins and sparrows have a lullaby-lilt to their songs. The pale blue sky of early spring spreads its arms of security around me. Even the angels are working overtime to protect my every step.

There is a tiny seed of life within me. God has chosen me to carry a minute bud of physical being and spiritual soul. A precious bit of forever. A child . A piece of eternity who will be part of me, part of his father, and part of all our ancestors for generations past. What a broad spectrum of genes and personality have culminated with pinpoint precision in the life of this new little soul. I am awed by the feeling that somehow I am in partnership with God. He has given me a special consignment from heaven.

I whisper the words again and again to myself. *A child. A baby.* In their new context they are words nearly incomprehensible. How can the miracle of this seed of life be taking place within me? But it is happening. I can feel its transformation taking hold of me.

I am still a child myself. And yet suddenly I feel I have been transformed from child

to woman

to mother.

It has not been simply a change from one to the next, but rather an addition of one to the others. God has taken incomplete portions of me to make me wholly as He intended woman to be from the beginning. The cycle is so wondrously complete that I can't help but wonder how I slipped so quietly from one stage to the next. It makes me want to stand outside myself and view this latest transformation from beginning to end.

And with this growing metamorphosis has come a change.

From ordinary
　　I've become glowingly beautiful.
From ordinary
　　I've been filled with tender awareness.
From ordinary
　　I've become deeply blessed!

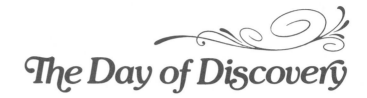

The Day of Discovery

The whole world suddenly seems pregnant! Everywhere I go my eyes are attracted to expectant mothers like metal to magnet. I never really noticed them before, and suddenly I see them standing on every street corner.

At the market I watch with envy the pear-shaped figures pushing their shopping carts. Some trudge wearily along behind their newly swollen tummies as they clumsily pick up cartons of low-fat milk and yogurt. Others seem to float gracefully by as they nonchalantly carry that special bundle under their hearts.

All have an almost ethereal glow about them — a peacefully soft light that plays about their eyes and mouths. As I gaze at their faces, I wonder if they feel as I do — that we are privileged to share a beautiful and special secret with God.

The secret of life. That basic genesis man for decades has tried and failed to duplicate in a test tube. A spark of life so fragile — yet strong enough to thrive in the rapidly developing fetus of a human being.

Like a portrait by an artist this little life has been conceived. It is an original. As if with separate strokes of the brush the Master Artist has made each individual cell completely unique. Never again will these same cells be united in quite the same way. This unborn child is already an original.

I clasp these secret thoughts to my heart and smile smugly to myself as I push my grocery cart past the frozen foods. I peek up at the mirror above the frozen peas. I can't help giggling at the reflection of the wide-eyed pregnant lady gazing back at me. That pregnant lady is me! I have the urge to stand on top of the frozen waffles and shout it to the world —

I'm going to be somebody's mother!

After all, I know no one can tell.
I just found out this morning.

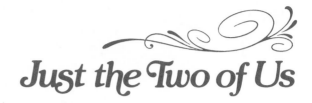

Just the Two of Us

Walking hand in hand in the fading evening light, we whisper only to the audience of each other with soft accents of laughter. Just the two of us. A silent squeeze of the palm says *I love you.*

The moon rises and the crisp dampness of nightfall descends upon us. We are two silhouettes painted by the fingers of moonlight reaching down through the shimmering leaves of a maple.

We pause a moment and breathe in the fragrance of spring. A gentle evening breeze stirs a thicket of lilacs laden heavily with spring's blossoms. Tenderly we are caressed by their sweet fragrance.

Lilacs and rosebuds. Baby's-breath and pale green fern. A floral bouquet reminiscent of our wedding. The soft fragrance of lilacs melts our memories into that special day. In the silence of the evening we can almost hear the velvet strains of the organ and picture the glowing candlelight upon the altar where we knelt. Just the two of us.

In a few months we will be three. But even in our intense excitement of expectancy it seems the tender joy of our just being two must stand still for a while.

Stand still? How long will it be before we become just two again — twenty years — twenty-five? When we are once again alone, will we be able to recapture this special feeling of these early years of marriage? Will we be too old (or too

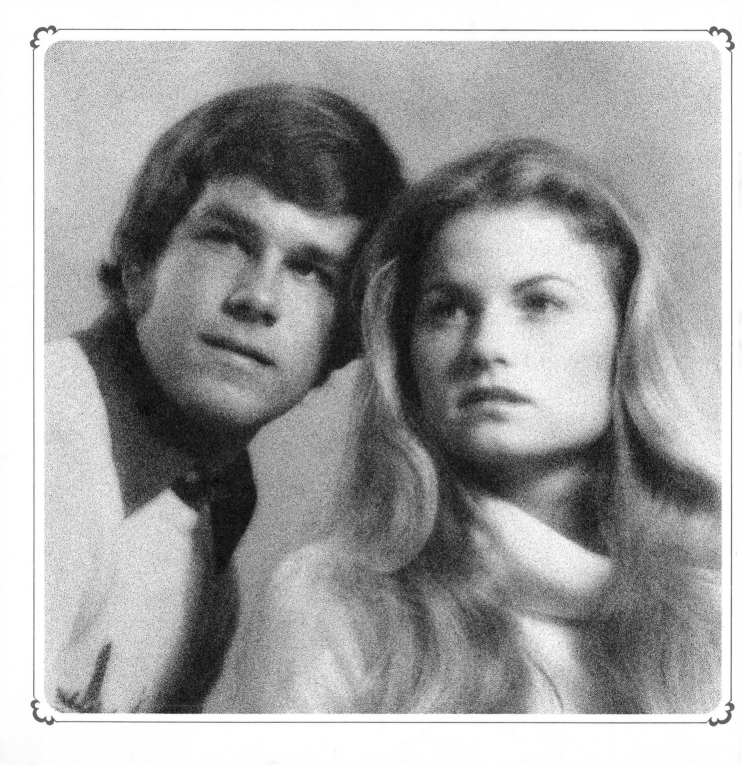

stuffy) to remember to once again
      walk arm in arm
                on a soft moonlit night?
      run barefoot through the hot sand at the beach,
             a fresh salty breeze stinging our faces?
      stay up half the night
             playing chess and eating peanuts?

Maybe — just maybe we won't need to wait twenty-five years to recapture these moments, but they must be nurtured to be kept alive. They may be forgotten like old clothes in a trunk if put aside for very long.

Even during our busy and delightful acceptance of the little one who is coming to make us three, or of those who may follow to make us four or five, we must set aside times to be just the two of us again. A refreshing time that will not rob our family of togetherness, but instead give us a sense of renewal to meet the demands of parenthood.

Once again our footsteps echo through the darkness. We continue our walk into the moonlight — and into the future. Like the sweet fragrance of the lilacs lingering in the breeze, we will remember our times of being just two long after these first gentle years are past. And with each fresh new experience of togetherness our love will blossom
      again.

I Am Fearfully & Wonderfully Made

*I*t's late at night, and I awaken with a start. Just a moment ago I felt the tiniest of flutters deep inside. The doctor said it could happen any time now. But surely this is my imagination. Wait! There it is again — just the faintest tap — tap — tap. I place my hand on the spot and wait for it to happen again. Moments tick by, and suddenly another gentle rapping comes from the inside, as softly as butterfly wings.

Excitedly I reach over and shake my sleeping husband. We must share this precious moment. Breathlessly we wait — and wait — and wait —. Wouldn't you know it — not a sign of anything. This little acrobat is exerting his independence already.

Drowsiness overtakes us, and we settle down to let sleep envelop once more. Before I drift into slumber, my thoughts turn with wonder to that little life growing inside. With his first gentle kick has come the knowledge that what I have been told and have accepted intellectually is physical reality. The cause of my woozy mornings and all-the-time-tired feeling is not a figment of my imagination!

A kick of reality. After just a few months of development, this miniature human being is completely formed — all organs in place and functioning. And he weighs just a little over one pound. He is even sporting the fuzziest bit of hair and has minute fingernails.

There is scientific proof that the human fetus sucks its thumb. I try to picture him and smile to myself in the dark. Just the thought of that thumb in his mouth somehow gives me an endearing glimpse of his coming personality.

As I contemplate the physical transformation that has taken place within me, I have a new appreciation for the psalmist's words:

You made all the delicate, inner parts of my body, and knit them together in my mother's womb. Thank you for making me so wonderfully complex! It is amazing to think about. Your workmanship is marvelous — and how well I know it. You were there while I was being formed in utter seclusion! You saw me before I was born and scheduled each day of my life before I began to breathe. Every day was recorded in your Book!

Psalm 139:13-17 (LB)

Another soft stirring of life warms my heart as I fall asleep.

The Glow of Sunlight in My Heart

*I*t is in this room that I feel so close to the reality of the child who will be. I sit on the floor, bending awkwardly over my expanding tummy as I carefully fold the tiny undershirts, nightgowns, and booties. I enjoy simply feeling their softness in my hands.

I've been here most of the afternoon. Folding and unfolding — and folding again. Placing the tiny items of clothing in the freshly lined drawer, then lifting them out again and holding them to my cheek. I examine each snap and button and tie the ribbons in bows.

I don't want to leave this sunny little room. With its fresh paint and bright new paper it looks as expectant as I do. A mobile hangs daintily over the crib. A bassinet covered in gingham and lace is settled snugly in the corner. Even the wooden rocker so lovingly made by daddy has its arms thrust forward in ready welcome.

All is in place and ready to welcome our child. Again I gently pick up a soft nightie, unsnap the fasteners and snap them again trying to imagine what the tiny being will be like who will be wearing it soon.

My imagination trips through the years, and I picture a little boy with eyes as clear and blue as the mountain sky. His hair plays around his ears like gold cotton candy. There is a rosy-tan glow to his face and a sunbeam in his eye —

Oh, for a child like this!

Then a freckle-faced imp comes skipping through my mind. One shoe is laced and the other is soiled and untied. He grins up at me mischievously and wrinkles his nose in glee. He carries my heart away with the frog in his pocket —

Oh, for a child like this!

A dainty little girl steps into the glow of my thoughts. Pink and sweet in ribbons and lace, she hums as she rocks her old-fashioned doll. Her long pigtails swing as she rocks to and fro. Large pensive eyes shyly smile up at me —

Oh, for a child like this!

An elfin-like creature with short cornsilk hair somersaults through my heart's door. Never still for a minute, she dances and sings and wiggles right into my arms. I can almost feel her kiss on my cheek —

Oh, for a child like this!

What will this child growing inside me be like? It's enchanting to think about the child who will be, but it really doesn't matter. Soon this little nightie I am holding so tenderly will be warmly wrapped around the soft pink body of my newborn child. A child unique in *every* way — custom-made in heaven for *us*. And my heart will be wrapped just as warmly with the joy of knowing that God has given me a child who will always send the glow of sunlight to my heart.

Oh, for a child like this!

I wonder what this child will turn out to be? For the hand of the Lord is surely upon him in some special way. Luke 1:66 (LB)

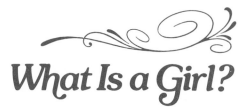

What Is a Girl?

*L*ittle girls are the nicest things that happen to people. They are born with a little bit of angel-shine about them, and though it wears thin sometimes, there is always enough left to lasso your heart — even when they are sitting in the mud, or crying temperamental tears, or parading up the street in mother's best clothes.

A little girl can be sweeter (and badder) oftener than anyone else in the world. She can jitter around, and stomp, and make funny noises that frazzle your nerves, yet just when you open your mouth, she stands there demure with that special look in her eyes. A girl is Innocence playing in the mud, Beauty standing on its head, and Motherhood dragging a doll by the foot.

Girls are available in five colors — black, white, red, yellow, or brown, yet Mother Nature always manages to select your favorite color when you place your order. They disprove the law of supply and demand — there are millions of little girls, but each is as precious as rubies.

God borrows from many creatures to make a little girl. He uses the song of a bird, the squeal of a pig, the stubbornness of a mule, the antics of a monkey, the spryness of a grasshopper, the curiosity of a cat, the speed of a gazelle, the slyness of a fox, the softness of a kitten, and to top it off He adds the mysterious mind of a woman.

A little girl likes new shoes, party dresses, small animals, first grade, noise makers, the girl next door, dolls, make-believe, dancing lessons, ice cream, kitchens, coloring books, make-up, cans of water, going visiting, tea parties, and one boy. She doesn't care so much for visitors, boys in general, large dogs, hand-me-downs, straight chairs, vegetables, snow-suits, or staying in the front yard. She is loudest when you are thinking, the prettiest when she has provoked you, the busiest at bedtime, the quietest when you want to show her off, and the most flirtatious when she absolutely must not get the best of you again.

Who else can cause you more grief, joy, irritation, satisfaction, embarrassment, and genuine delight than this combination of Eve, Salome, and Florence Nightingale? She can muss up your home, your hair, and your dignity — spend your money, your time, and your temper — then just when your patience is ready to crack, her sunshine peeks through and you've lost again.

Yes, she is a nerve-racking nuisance, just a noisy bundle of mischief. But when your dreams tumble down and the world is a mess — when it seems you are pretty much of a fool after all — she can make you a king when she climbs on your knee and whispers, "I love you best of all!"

Alan Beck

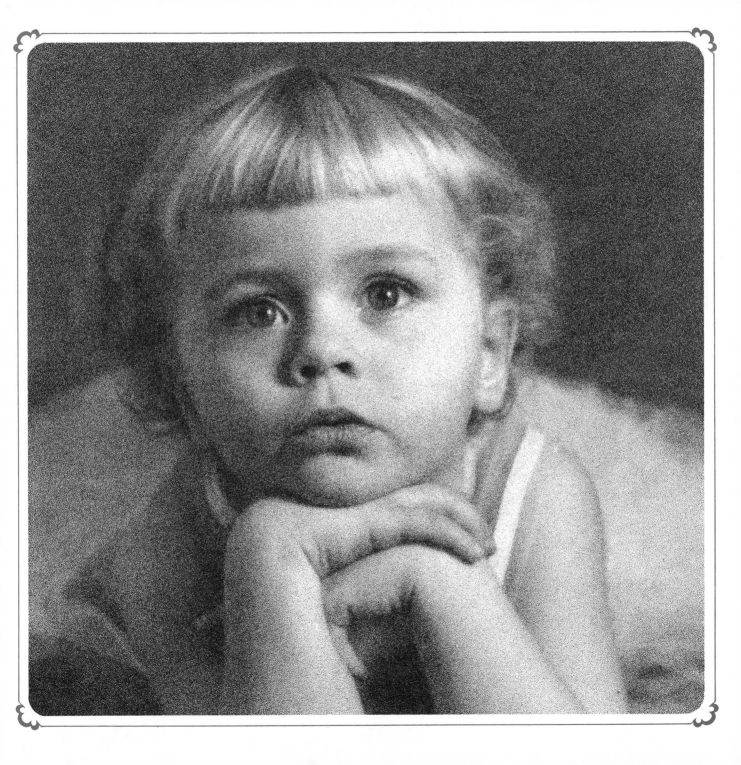

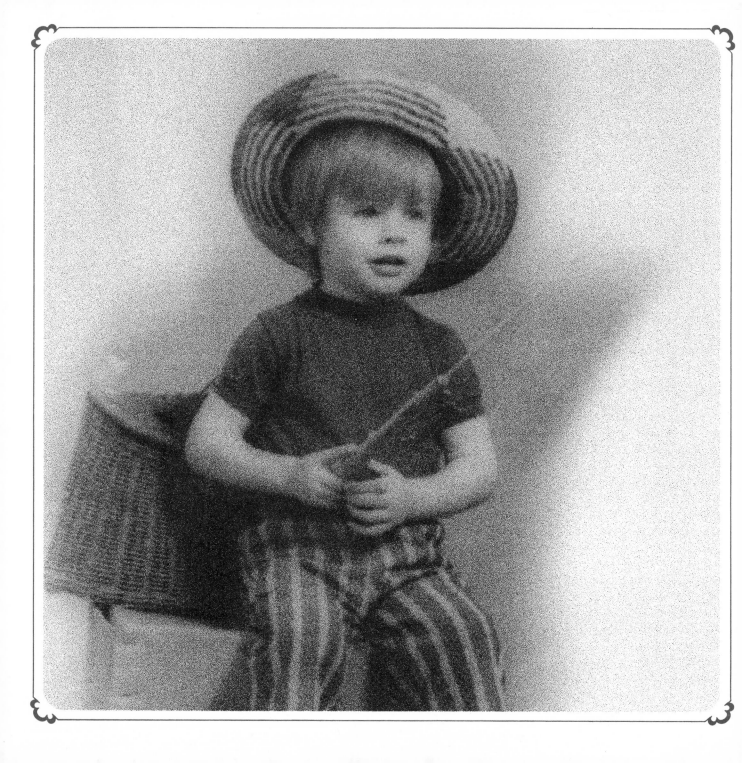

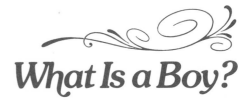

What Is a Boy?

*B*etween the innocence of babyhood and the dignity of manhood we find a delightful creature called a boy. Boys come in assorted sizes, weights, and colors, but all boys have the same creed: To enjoy every second of every minute of every hour of every day and to protest with noise (their only weapon) when their last minute is finished and the adult males pack them off to bed at night.

Boys are found everywhere — on top of, underneath, inside of, climbing on, swinging from, running around, or jumping to. Mothers love them, little girls hate them, older sisters and brothers tolerate them, adults ignore them, and Heaven protects them. A boy is Truth with dirt on its face, Beauty with a cut on its finger, Wisdom with bubble gum in its hair, and the Hope of the future with a frog in its pocket.

When you are busy, a boy is an inconsiderate, bothersome, intruding jangle of noise. When you want him to make a good impression, his brain turns to jelly or else he becomes a savage, sadistic, jungle creature bent on destroying the world and himself with it.

A boy is a composite — he has the appetite of a horse, the digestion of a sword swallower, the energy of a pocket-size atomic bomb, the curiosity of a cat, the lungs of a dictator, the imagination of a Paul Bunyan, the shyness of a violet, the audacity of a steel trap, the enthusiasm of a firecracker, and when he makes something he has five thumbs on each hand.

He likes ice cream, knives, saws, Christmas, comic books, the boy across the street, woods, water (in its natural habitat), large animals, Dad, trains, Saturday mornings, and fire engines. He is not much for Sunday school, company, schools, books without pictures, music lessons, neckties, barbers, girls, overcoats, adults, or bedtime.

Nobody else is so early to rise, or so late to supper. Nobody else gets so much fun out of trees, dogs, and breezes. Nobody else can cram into one pocket a rusty knife, a half-eaten apple, three feet of string, an empty Bull Durham sack, two gum drops, six cents, a slingshot, a chunk of unknown substance, and a genuine super-sonic code ring with a secret compartment.

A boy is a magical creature — you can lock him out of your workshop, but you can't lock him out of your heart. You can get him out of your study, but you can't get him out of your mind. Might as well give up — he is your captor, your jailer, your boss, and your master — a freckle-faced, pint-sized, cat-chasing bundle of noise. But when you come home at night with only the shattered pieces of your hopes and dreams, he can mend them like new with the two magic words — "Hi Dad!"

Alan Beck

Letter to My Unborn Child - From Daddy

*H*i, Little Fella!

There is a brand-new pathway leading to my heart. And on this path softly treads a child — you. The gently awakening reality of *you!*

I've watched you growing day by day, becoming stronger with each rippling kick and scooting jab under your mother's ribs. You've been a living reality to her from the very beginning, carried just under her heart.

With me it's a little different. Becoming a father is happening *to* me, not *within* me. The miracle of your life is stepping up to the threshold of my heart, and your reality will step through my heart's door the moment I reach out and touch you for the first time. As your birth so quickly approaches, I am awed and a little frightened by the growing sense of responsibility that faces me — the grave responsibility of parenthood. It is taking God only nine months to make you, but it will take me a lifetime to learn to be a parent.

I saw a picture once of a father walking along a smooth and quiet beach close to the water where the soft, silty sand stretched for miles. He left large, striding footprints in the sand. Behind him walked a child — skipping and hopping from one large print to the next — trying to step in each of his father's footsteps.

As I think about this picture, it frightens me a little. I don't know if my footprints will be large enough or clear enough for you to follow throughout your life. I know that as much as my love for you will grow, I still will not begin to fill all your needs. My footprints alone will be inadequate.

But there is Someone whose footprints leave a perfect path. A path that will never fail you. For on this path are the footprints of

perfect love —

> *tender and compassionate,*

perfect peace —

> *gentle and calm,*

perfect joy —

> *blessed and radiant,*

footprints that are unchanging and endless. These footprints are imprinted with clarity and are outlined in truth. They once led to Calvary and can now lead you along the path of life.

Step through my heart's door, my little one, and I will take your tiny baby hand in mine and hold it firmly as we begin our journey as father and child.

A journey in the reflection of His love —

> following the footprints leading to the door of eternity.

Letter to My Unborn Child - From Mommy

*D*earest Little One,

My happiness is tinged with just a hint of sadness. You have been an integral part of me for nearly nine months. You are a separate and complete human being, and yet because you have been conceived and so carefully nurtured within me, I cannot help but feel a little melancholy as the day of your birth approaches.

But this hint of mist in my heart will be dispersed by joy as I hold you in my arms and welcome you into our world.

Our world, and the special place in it where you belong — a special place snug in my arms.

Then clutching tightly to my hand.

Then lingering a bit as you toddle around.

Then walking away —

a little farther at a time.

All the while discovering the way to your own little corner of the world.

A beautiful place where you'll

hear a lullaby sung softly,

hold a drop of rain in your hand,
touch the fragile petal of a flower with your nose,
catch a snowflake on your tongue,
pick a wild blackberry on a hot and dusty day
      and feel its warm burst of delight in your mouth.

All for the first time!

For you see, you've done nothing before. Everything you experience, whether it be doing, seeing, hearing, or feeling, will be for the very first time.

What a great adventure you have in store as you begin your own unique journey through life! A journey of discovery in a brand-new world. A world that can be beautiful or plain, exciting or dull, full of adventure or empty. What your world becomes will be up to you as you reach out to grasp it.

And so, my little one, I hold out my hand with the whole world in it. It's yours, you know. Because already

you belong.

The Gentle Whisper of Wisdom

I'm scared!

Not of becoming a mother (so far that part seems easy), but of *being* a mother. And not just *a* mother, but the *best* mother I have the wisdom and knowledge to be.

And that's the part that frightens me! Where am I suddenly supposed to discover this source of motherly wisdom and discernment? What lies beyond the months ahead when a great deal more is demanded of me than simply watching for signs of hunger and changing wet diapers?

When this challenge of the future faces me —

Will my answers be the right ones?

Will my decisions be wise?

Will I suddenly lift an unopened curtain in my mind to find Wisdom sweetly smiling at me?

A verse steals softly through the maze of my questioning mind — a gentle whisper from God bringing peace and calm assurance.

But the wisdom that comes from heaven is first of all pure and full of quiet gentleness. Then it is peace-loving and courteous. It allows discussion and is willing to yield to others; it is full of mercy and good deeds. It is wholehearted and straightforward and sincere.

James 3:17 (LB)

Our child's life comes to us as an empty vessel waiting to be filled. Each crystal drop of wisdom — whether it be right or wrong — dropped into this vessel melts into the content of our child's life, there to remain forever.

That in itself is an incredible responsibility. But the beauty of it is that the wisdom we seek for filling this precious vessel *does* have a Source. A Source that is

pure

full of quiet gentleness

peace-loving

courteous

full of mercy and good deeds

wholehearted
straightforward
sincere.

What greater wisdom can there be?

Oh, Lord, thank You for the wisdom in Your Word. Thank You for being the Source of that wisdom. I am no longer afraid. I am not alone as I open the door of motherhood. I know that the gentle whisper of Your divine and all-discerning wisdom is there for me to hear — if I will but listen.

Perfect Love Casts Out Fear

I sought the Lord, and he answered me,
and delivered me from all my fears.
Look to him, and be radiant;
so your faces shall never be ashamed.[1]

We live within the shadow of the Almighty,
sheltered by the God who is above all gods.
This I declare, that he alone is my refuge,
my place of safety;
He is my God, and I am trusting Him.
He will shield you with his wings!
They will shelter you.
His faithful promises are your armor.

Now you don't need to be afraid of the dark any more,
nor fear the dangers of the day.
For he orders his angels to protect you
wherever you go.
They will steady you with their hands
to keep you from stumbling.[2]

Fear not, for I am with you.
Do not be dismayed.
I am your God.
    I will strengthen you;
       I will help you;
          I will uphold you with my victorious right hand.
I am holding you by your right hand —
    I, the Lord your God —
    and I say to you,
       Don't be afraid;
        I am here to help you. [3]

For God hath not given us the spirit of fear;
    but of power,
       and of love,
         and of a sound mind. [4]

Lord, as I approach my time of childbirth, I have natural fears and apprehensions of the unknown that lies ahead of me.

I have prepared myself for this moment the best I humanly can. But I ask You to take complete control where my human weakness ends and Your strength and courage begin.

May I feel the tenderness of Your love as its warmth surrounds me in my hour of need, for I know Your perfect love will leave no room for my fear.

[1]Psalm 34:4-5 (RSV)

[2]Psalm 91:1-2, 4-5, 11-12 (LB)

[3]Isaiah 41:10, 13 (LB)

[4]2 Timothy 1:7 (KJV)

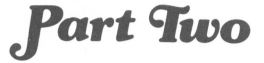

Part Two

"*For this child I prayed.*"

— *1 Samuel 1:27* (KJV)

Birth

Just when each bud was big with bloom,
And as prophetic of perfume,
When spring, with her bright horoscope,
Was sweet as an unuttered hope;

Just when the last star flickered out,
And twilight, like a soul in doubt,
Hovered between the dark and dawn,
And day lay waiting to be born;

Just when the gray and dewy air
Grew sacred as an unvoiced prayer,
And somewhere through the dusk she heard
The stirring of a nested bird —

Four angels gloried the place:
Wan Pain unveiled her awful face;
Joy, soaring, sang; Love, brooding, smiled;
Peace laid upon her breast a child.

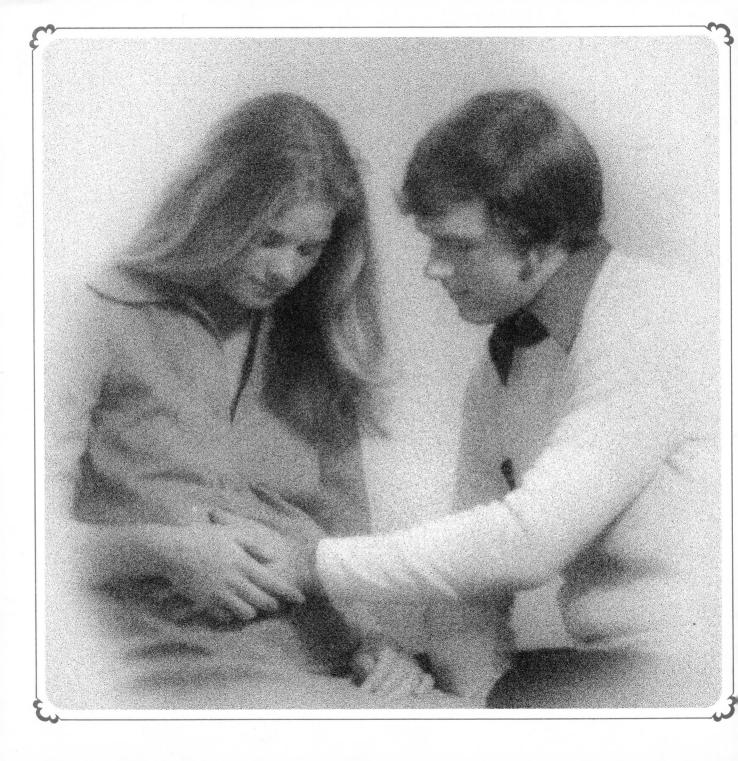

Entering the Circle of Creation

I am Eve.

I am woman.

I am created.

I am creation.

I am as old as creation itself — yet as young as the child within me.

I step into the circle of creation as a part of its beginning and a part of its continuum —

for I am the door through which another unique life shall enter the circle.

I stand in the center of an intense spectrum of God's love. At this moment, I am the most precious jewel of all His humanity. The warmth of His love fills every corner of my being, chasing out all traces of apprehension and fear. For you see —

my time has begun.

A tightening and tingling sensation slowly spreads across my abdomen. It is growing stronger than those before. I reach for my husband's hand and bask in the strength and encouragement I see written on his face. As the contraction moves toward its peak, I close my eyes and concentrate on my breathing. Like a small boat upon the sea, I ride with the swelling wave. As it ebbs, I float lazily and await the next rippling swirl.

I rest my hands lightly across my stomach, spreading my fingers to feel the ripened bones of my child. Soon this house will be empty, and my child will have a new home in my arms. I can't help but give those bumps of elbows and knees a loving little pat, for I know that within minutes I will touch them again — without a wall of flesh between. I will know that what is an elbow is really an elbow — not the maybes of a foot or knee as in the guessing games of recent weeks.

Another contraction begins. The intensity of it shakes my calm resolutions. It is a strange feeling — almost as if I am not in control of my own body. Like an outside force is the cause and the effect.

I am not afraid. Rather than fear, I feel a breath of excitement and a keen sense of anticipation. With each billowing wave of pain I rejoice, knowing I am that much closer to holding the reality of God's creation in my arms — the warm body of my newborn child.

> *It will be the same joy as that of a woman in labor when her child is born — her anguish gives place to rapturous joy and the pain is forgotten. You have sorrow now, but I will see you again and then you will rejoice and no one can rob you of that joy.*
> *John 16:21-22 (LB)*

To Be Intertwined There Forever

My journey toward joy is at an end. I can see the light at the end of the long, dark tunnel. The brilliance of the light nearly blinds me. I look up and smile. The light at the end of my tunnel is merely the spotlight over the delivery table.

The discomfort of the past hours dreamily disappears and pushes itself past my consciousness to be forgotten forever. I lie back limp and totally exhausted. Yet somehow I am encompassed by exhilaration and great pride. I have stepped over the threshold of motherhood.

My child is born! *My child. My child!* I whisper the words again and again to my swelling heart. During these first precious moments of her life she begins to wrap herself around my soul — to be intertwined there forever. I gaze at her with fascination — her little fists waving so indignantly in the air — her pink pixie brow wrinkling itself in preparation for a loud and gusty cry — her tiny round toes (a miniature replica of her daddy's) wiggling as she kicks.

Mere words cannot express her newborn beauty. It's a beauty completely alien to the word as I have always known it. A beauty that does not rest on comeliness, but in the nucleus of the entire being. A beauty reflecting the very face of God.

She is His creation.

His image.

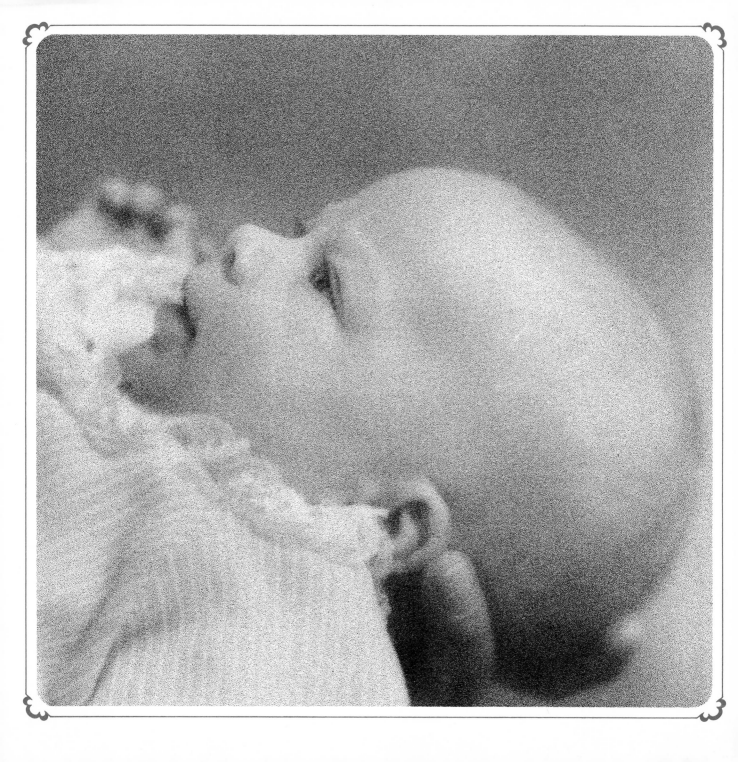

This is the absolute of her life — the whole of her being. What total worth He has given this helpless infant! What a blanket of binding love He has tenderly wrapped around her!

I reach out to touch her for the first time. As I feel the soft, wet warmth of her skin, it seems I am touching the very breath of God. I am touching a tiny miracle of life — and the center of creation.

All of this is *my child* . . .

my child . . .

my child!

The Little Princess in Bassinet No. 3

Hi there, little princess!

It's your daddy! (I'm the one tapping on the nursery glass with a football under one arm and a toy airplane under the other.)

Don't laugh.

I know it seems kind of dumb, but until just a little while ago I thought you were a boy. (After all, that's what the doctor and two nurses told us!)

Hey! You're beautiful — you really are. Even with your scrunched-up nose and bright pink face. And look at those long tapered fingers — you'd have made a great quarterback. By the way, what do you think about taking flying lessons?

Oh, wow! Is that a smile?

I wish you would open your eyes for a minute. (My goodness, you mind well for being only an hour old.) They're dark blue and absolutely beautiful. I can see you're going to take after your daddy.

Why is everyone smiling at me? Their faces light up every time I tap on the glass and wave to you.

Hey! Another smile!

What personality already!

Little girl, you and your daddy are going to have some great times ahead. A daughter is something pretty wonderful! And I'm just beginning to find out about a special place that's been reserved for you in my heart. A place that's warm and cozy and just the right size for a brand-new baby daughter.

Hey, little princess in Bassinet No. 3 —

I LOVE YOU!

A Song of Praise

"Sir, do you remember me?" Hannah asked him. "I am the woman who stood here that time praying to the Lord! I asked him to give me this child, and he has given me my request; and now I am giving him back to the Lord for as long as he lives." So she left him there at the Tabernacle for the Lord to use.

This was Hannah's prayer:

"How I rejoice in the Lord!
How he has blessed me!

. . . . .

For the Lord has solved my problem.
How I rejoice!
No one is as holy as the Lord!
There is no other God,
Nor any Rock like our God."

1 Samuel 1:26-28; 2:1-2 (LB)

And now at long last I hold my child in my arms. It is only hours since her birth, but in my drowsy off- and-on-again sleep it seems like days — and my arms have ached to hold her.

She comes to me with a tiny bow scotch-taped to her fuzzy head, placed there by a fun-loving nurse. I slowly unwrap the tightly secured blanket from around her to inspect her fingers and toes. She objects loudly, and I clumsily

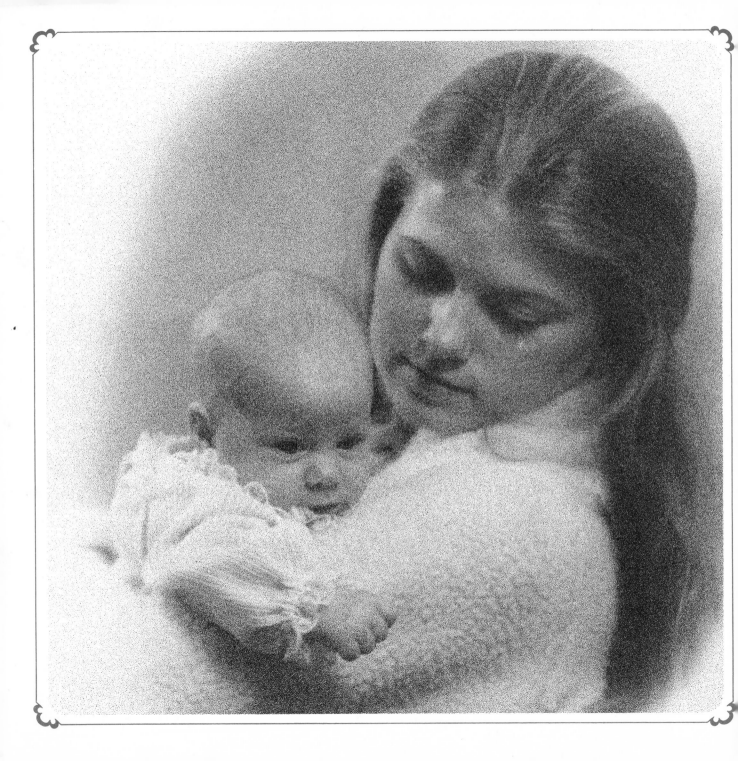

rewrap her as fast as I can — my fumbling fingers and hands not quite knowing where to do what.

I settle back into my bed and hold her against me. Unexpected emotion wells up inside me as I comfort her for the first time. Her tiny sobs subside, and joy fills my heart.

My thoughts turn to Hannah, the mother of baby Samuel of long ago. How she agonized during those long, barren years while she prayed for a child! What all-supreme joy and tender emotion she must have felt as she held her baby boy in her arms for the first time. No wonder she prayed such a prayer of praise and thanksgiving to the Lord.

With the warmth of my child in my arms at last, I, too, find my heart lifting in spontaneous praise to the Lord for the answer to my heart's longing and His goodness to me —

Shout with joy before the Lord, O earth!
Obey him gladly;
Come before him,
singing with joy.
. . . .
He made us — we are his people,
    the sheep of his pasture.
Go through his open gates with great thanksgiving;
Enter his courts with praise.
Give thanks to him and bless his name.
For the Lord is always good.
He is always loving and kind,
And his faithfulness goes on and on
    to each succeeding generation.

Psalm 100 (LB)

Prayer of Dedication

*"And now I am giving him back
to the Lord for as long as he lives."*
1 Samuel 1:28 (LB)

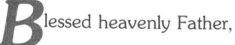lessed heavenly Father,

We kneel today at the same altar where we knelt before You in holy matrimony a few years ago. Today we bring before You the fruit of our union — the very essence of our love for each other.

You have richly blessed us by giving us this child to love. We know that "every good and perfect gift is from above," and we thank You for the blessed gift of this new life.

As we bring our child to You, we also present ourselves. Create in us a clean heart and renew a right spirit within us as we lead her through the years she will be entrusted to us. May we look to You for guidance and wisdom as we lead her through this uncertain world. May her world be firm and secure as it is grounded in Your love.

From Your Word we know that nothing is closer to Your heart than a little child. For You said:

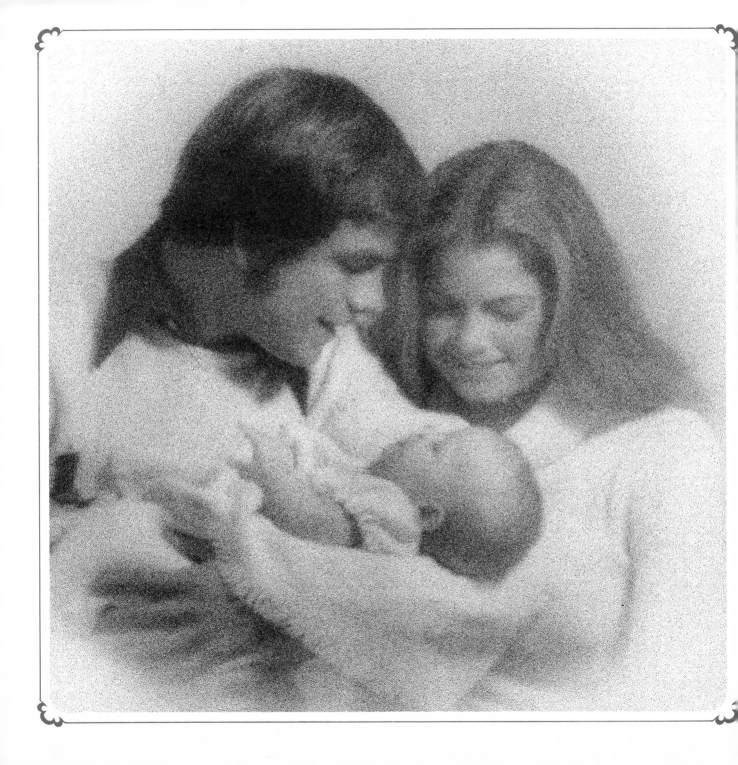

"Anyone who humbles himself as this little child, is the greatest in the Kingdom of Heaven."

Matthew 18:4 (LB)

Help us never to stop learning the lessons of humility, love, and trust from our child. May she be a constant reminder of the sacredness and preciousness of life itself.

You placed supreme importance on the life of a child when You said, "Let the children come to Me."

Therefore, we bring our child to You.
We dedicate her for Your glory, Your service,
and the joy of Your love and fellowship.
May Your grace be manifested in her life.
Breathe upon her very soul.
Touch her with Your love.
We lift our child heavenward and give her back to You.
Carry her forever as a little lamb
in Your arms.

You've Grown Up So Quickly It Seems

A frilly bassinet graces the corner with its brand-new guest of honor nestled snug and secure among the ruffles and lace. We arrived home from the hospital this morning, and the precious bundle who rests in that interior is only three days old.

I can't keep my eyes off her. At the slightest excuse of a tiny burp or soft cry I rush over to peek through the lace at the little angel who has come to make her home in our hearts.

I lie down on the bed next to the bassinet to get more much-needed rest while she sleeps so peacefully. If I listen carefully, I can hear her soft and shallow breathing.

For the hundredth time since we arrived home, I can't resist the temptation. I tiptoe over to the bassinet and peer in. Her delicate pink petal face is framed by the tiny yellow rosebuds on her nightie. I reach down and rest my fingertips on her tightly clinched fist. Her skin is as soft as a rose petal. As I gaze down at her, the lines of a haunting poem slip through my mind.

Dreams Do Come True

Daughter of mine, little daughter of
mine,
You've grown up so quickly it seems;
Ah, sure and 'twas only yesterday
You were just a part of my dreams,

I dreamed of a daughter with soft brown
curls
And eyes of delphinium blue;
I dreamed of the hours we'd spend in
play
Of the many things we'd do.

I dreamed of the moments of joy we'd
share,
The secrets — just you and I —
Mother and daughter, daughter and
mother,
Together as the days passed by.

But daughter of mine, little daughter of
mine,
You've grown up so quickly it seems;
Ah, sure and 'twas only yesterday
You were just a part of my dreams.

PHYLLIS C. MICHAEL

In my imagination, I picture her as the years rush by so quickly —

There she is, pigtails and freckles, all dressed up for her first day of school . . . and here she comes in her cap and gown, smiling proudly as she tramps across the platform to receive her diploma . . . I look again and she is floating down the aisle on her daddy's arm, angelic in an aura of white lace . . . and there she is again, cuddling a baby just three days old. Daughter of mine, little daughter of mine, you've grown up so quickly it seems. . . .

Gladly I am snatched back into the reality of now by a soft, gurgling cry. Fuzzy blue eyes open and gaze unseeingly up at me, searching for comfort. Tenderly I reach down and pick up that sweet bundle of blankets and baby. As I lie down again, I hold her close — close enough for her to hear that familiar rhythm of my heartbeat and breathing.

Contentedly she snuggles close with her head upon my breast, and with the tiniest of sighs her big blue eyes close. I, too, close my eyes in silent prayer, asking God to let me always fully enjoy and appreciate each precious moment of her tomorrows before this little seedling turns into a sunflower.

Cold Feet & a Warm Heart

Our brand-new alarm clock sounds off at precisely 2:14 A.M.! A hungry little howl grows louder and louder.

I slide through the grogginess of a sound sleep, gradually becoming aware that I must exchange this heavenly warm bed for the cold feet of a middle-of-the-night feeding. I groan and shiver and grope for my slippers. (It seems I never can find them in the dark!)

By the time I reach the nursery I'm wide-awake and looking forward to a blessed time of quietness with my hungry little bundle of love — a time of deep thought and quiet devotion with just the Lord, my child, and me (and a steaming hot cup of tea).

With such full and busy days, my spirit yearns for the peace and quiet of the small hours of the morning. It is a time of renewal with spiritual food for the strength I need tomorrow, just as my child is renewed physically by the warm nourishment she receives from me.

I settle back into the rocker with my precious babe at my breast, gently rocking to the sweet music of her contentment. As she gulps hungrily, soft scooting sounds from deep in her throat rise and fall rhythmically. With these gentle notes as background music my thoughts turn to other mothers — knowing that almost every mother who ever lived must surely have held her child in her arms and listened to that same sweet voice of contentment in the dark of the night. Did they ponder the same special and secret thoughts I hold so dear?

I think about Mary, Jesus' mother; she has become a real person to me since the beauty of childbirth dawned in my being. It's as if her experience has in some mysterious way become part of mine. What sublime importance is placed upon my motherhood when I think about it being second only to hers!

I read her song of joy with a greater depth of understanding.

> Oh, how I praise the Lord.
> How I rejoice in God my Savior!
> For he took notice of his lowly servant girl,
> And now generation after generation
>   forever shall call me blest of God.
> For he, the mighty Holy One, has done
>   great things to me.
> His mercy goes on from generation to generation,
>   to all who reverence him.
>
> *Luke 1:46-50 (LB)*

Her praise to the Lord came before she even saw her child or snuggled Him to her breast for the first time. If she was so filled with joy beforehand, can you imagine how she felt when God incarnate lay in her arms? Jesus — the Son of God!

With love-filled eyes I gaze down at my child, feeling the indescribable joy of her existence. I feel a warm rush of kinship with that young Hebrew mother. I don't know what her thoughts were in the middle of the night as she tenderly rocked and fed her child, but I wonder if her songs of praise and prayers of adoration were like mine.

A Touch o' the Blues

*I will comfort you there as a little one
is comforted by its mother.*

Isaiah 66:13 *(LB)*

One end after the other! I feed one end, and a few moments later the other end needs attention. Somehow the aesthetic beauty of motherhood seems far away.

What has happened to that proud and joyful countenance I had even yesterday? I feel so overpowered by the drudgery involved in my new role. It's much more than I expected! A full-time job was never like this. At least when I was working I was able to leave after putting in my eight hours. But where can I go now? I'm trapped in wall-to-wall diapers!

With a few stinging tears of self-pity beginning to slip into my eyes, I glance around the living room and into the kitchen. There are dozens of diapers piled high on the sofa waiting to be folded. The breakfast dishes are still on the table with the faint, lingering aroma of bacon. On the kitchen sink a plastic baby bathtub is prominently displayed with towels, jars of baby lotion, powder, and cotton balls scattered here and there.

I look down at my housecoat and slippers. It's almost noon, and there's been no time to get dressed and comb my hair. I sink into an easy chair and wonder if I'll ever have time for myself again.

And wouldn't you know it — just as I lean back and relax I hear a tiny, muffled wail from around the corner and down the hall. Tears begin to trickle down my cheeks. I feel so unappreciated and unrewarded for giving myself 100 percent to the task of motherhood.

There is a label for my feelings — post-partum depression — or the plain ol' baby blues. But it makes me a little angry to think what I feel has a label. It makes me seem a little less individual, and it doesn't really help to know "everybody goes through it." I can't help smiling, though, at my indignation during such an enjoyable time of self-pity.

Quietness once again drifts through the house. I tiptoe to the nursery, and tranquillity floods my soul as my eyes rest upon that delicate bundle with her eyes closed in peaceful sleep. As I stand over her, I think of the words of Jesus:

> *Anyone who takes care of a little child like this is caring for me! And whoever cares for me is caring for God who sent me. Your care for others is the measure of your greatness.* Luke 9:48 *(LB)*

What was I just saying about feeling unappreciated and unrewarded? Suddenly I am overwhelmed by the knowledge that in caring for this babe of mine *I am actually caring for Jesus Himself!* What a wondrously emancipating thought! He loves this little infant so much that when I perform the mundane tasks that motherhood demands — I am actually caring for Him.

Motherhood has new value — that of

utmost value.

Just a Quick Hug Away

A tender, fleeting glimpse of a smile makes its debut, then disappears. Is it real — or just another gas bubble in the tummy? It comes again and lingers for a bit. This time I know for sure!

It's a cloudy winter's morning, but the light from her first smile creates an indescribable glow in the room. She is hearing her first songs about Jesus. I sing "Jesus Loves Me" joyously louder as I watch that tiny face peering into mine. I don't ever want to stop singing to her. My eyes are misty as I bow my head and thank the Lord for the unexpected joy of that first smile.

It saddens me to think that this precious moment could have been lost to me. What if I hadn't been here? What if I had yielded to the temptation that's been tickling the back of my mind since I decided on motherhood in exchange for a career? It seems that voices all around are becoming a chorus, nearly shouting that a woman's "fulfillment" can only be found outside the home. This may be true for some. But for me — I'd rather not miss out on the joy and fulfillment that's right in front of my eyes — the unfolding of a little miracle.

What if I had missed that first smile? There will be others, but how can these joyous moments of her first smile ever be duplicated?

I want to watch firsthand the world debut of the tiny life God has given me. I want to be with her as all of her firsts open as morning-glories in sunlight.

To be the one
She reaches for first —
To hear her first chortling giggle —
To be the one
She stumbles toward as she takes those
      first wobbly steps —
To receive the first crumpled dandelion
      she picks!

As she grows and explores this new world of hers, I want to be just a quick hug away. These years of discovery are so short. The years of independence will overtake her all too quickly. My time of rediscovering the world through her eyes will soon be over.

But for now — there is a whole universe awaiting her discovery.

In the Basket of His Love

The sunlight reflects sparkling prisms of light dancing across the swirling blue-green water. A dark-haired woman stands with her baby at the river's edge, a light breeze brushing against her face like a warm caress. But she can't help shivering in the bright morning sun. She knows what lies ahead.

She gazes down at the tiny bundle in her arms with a full and aching heart. Her baby boy is only three months old. He is the joy and delight of her life. His dark curly hair and luminous brown eyes make her heart skip a beat as he smiles up at her.

Holding him close to her pounding heart, she wonders how anyone could possibly want to harm him. It doesn't seem possible — but he is in the gravest danger. His very life is at stake.

There is a plan to save his life, but so many things could go wrong. She looks down at the basket at her feet. Fear spreads its icy fingers around her heart as she thinks of placing her beloved child in that basket and releasing it into the cold, dark water.

She prays for faith that God will take care of her child. She whispers again and again to herself that God loves her little boy more than she does and that He will endlessly care for him. Suddenly the chill she felt is gone — the warmth of the sun seeps through to her very soul, and she rejoices in knowing she is no longer

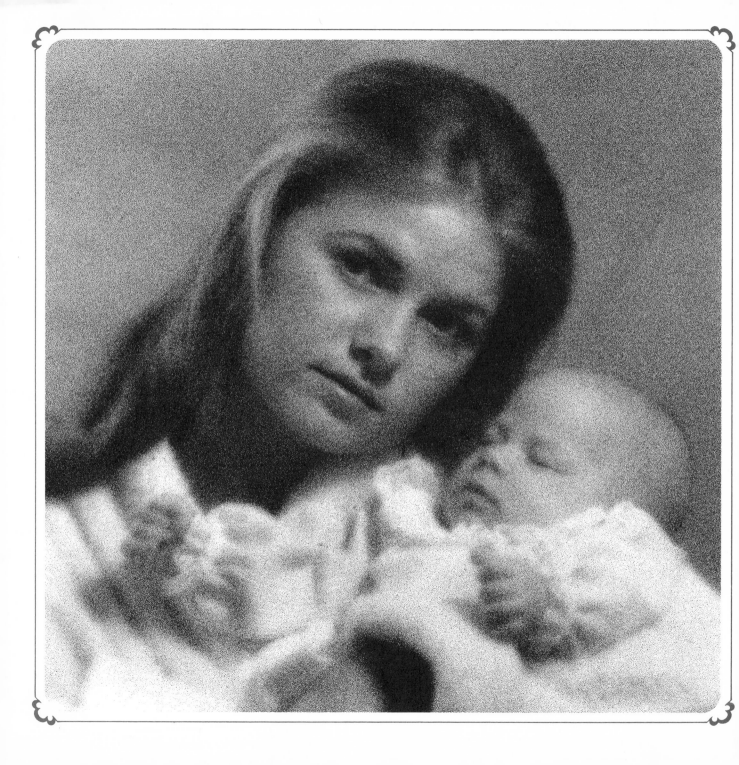

alone. Her terror disappears like an early morning mist in the light of the rising sun.

With new strength she spreads the blankets and places her precious infant in the basket. He chuckles softly as she gently tucks the covers around his tiny warm body. Quick tears spring to her eyes as she kisses his rosy cheek and places the lid on the basket. Still hearing soft coos inside, she kneels at the water's edge and relinquishes her child into the infinite love and care of his heavenly Father.

> *O God of little Moses, I know You are the same yesterday, today, and forever — that Your love for my child is just as strong as it was for baby Moses; that You have a plan for her life just as You did for his. Your total love for her erases my worries and fears about her tomorrows; they are all in Your hands. Help me have the wisdom and strength of Moses' mother so that I may place this tender little life in the basket of Your love — and leave her there for now and forever.*

A Chain Reaction of Love

*L*ove can slip around the corner and into your heart on a warm spring day, as romantic and sunny as a mountain meadow covered with a purple-blue carpet of bachelor's buttons. The lilting joy of a first love!

Love can begin as a seed planted by caring parents, watered and nurtured, until at last it bursts forth in full growth. The love freely given by a mother and father.

Love can be as warm and homey as sipping a cup of tea by a cozy fire, chatting about anything and everything with a special friend. The love wrapped in the warmth of friendship.

The greatest love of all can quench the thirst of a searching heart in the form no other love takes, the compassionate and all-encompassing love of our heavenly Father! The Source of love.

A new love has quietly formed in my heart — I am a mother. And I have a child to love! What began as a tiny tickle in my heart, even before she was born, has yawned and stretched its arms out in my soul, awakening that innate something within me called motherly love.

Love begets love. It is only because we are first loved that we are able to love. God made us that way. This is even the way His love for us works: we love Him because He first loved us.

A mother's love is like that, too. It creates a reservoir within us that throughout our lives becomes deeper and deeper as it is filled with love. Later it becomes so deep that the love it holds is endless. It is ready to spill over and flow into another little life — to begin building another channel to fill with love. A chain reaction of love.

A mother's love is not constantly the same. It changes and it grows. The forms it takes are boundless. It can be found in

gentle strength

sweet serenity

quiet peacefulness

Comforting arms

echoes of merriment

and shades of exasperation!

It somehow molds itself to fit every special moment shared by a mother and her child.

How like this love must be our heavenly Father's love for us. Being a mother somehow gives me a new sense of the depth and breadth of His love for me, His child.

Maybe this is how God intended for my child to learn about His love for her. My deep and tender love as her mother is but a reflection of a much greater love, a perfect love, that she will only be able to begin to comprehend much later.

Part Three

"*Children are a gift from God; they are his reward.*"

— *Psalm 127:3 (LB)*

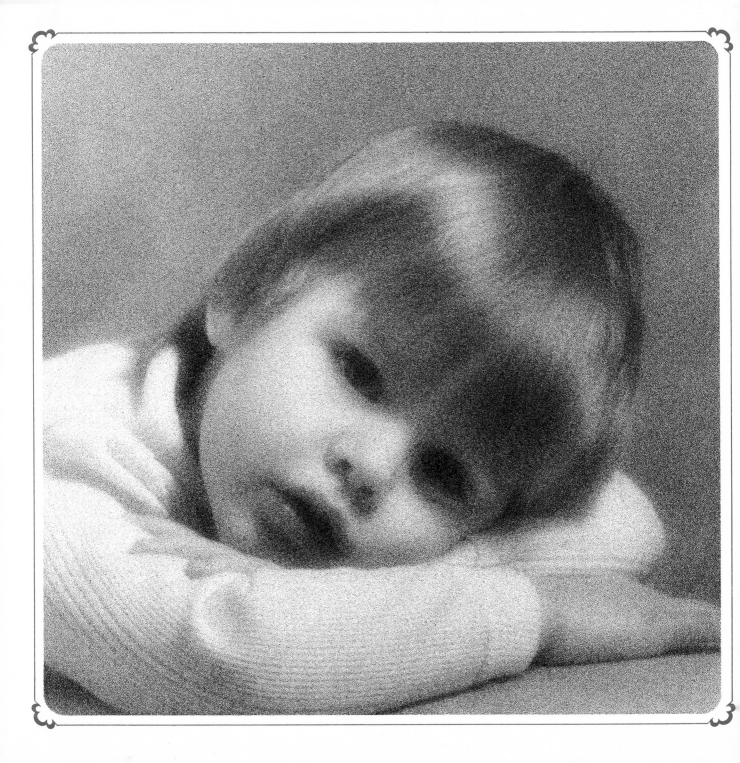

A Tribute to Childhood

When God made the child, He began early in the morning. He watched the golden hues of the rising day chasing away the darkness, and He chose the azure of the opening heavens for the color of childhood's eyes, the crimson of the clouds to paint its cheeks, and the gold of the morning for its flowing tresses. He listened to the song of the birds as they sang and warbled and whispered, and strung childhood's harp with notes now soft and low — now sweet and strong.

He saw little lambs among the flock romp and play and skip, and He put play into childhood's heart. He saw the silvery brook and listened to its music and He made the laughter of the child like the ripple of the brook. He saw angels of light as upon the wings of love they hastened to holy duty, and He formed the child's heart in purity and love.

And having made the child, He sent it out to bring joy into the home, laughter on the green, and gladness everywhere. He sent it into the home and said to the parents, "Nourish and bring up this child for Me." He sent it to the state and said, "Deal tenderly with it, and it will bless and not curse you." He sent it to the nation and said, "Be good to the child. It is thy greatest asset and thy hope."

George W. Rideout

A Bouquet of Sunshine

Sunshine floods the room and creates a speckled pattern of shining patches on the floor. With her cheeks rosy from a late afternoon nap, she rubs her eyes and blinks at the bright surprise. Her funny little toddle turns into a run as she hurries toward the nearest spot of sunshine. She stoops down and touches the spot only to see it disappear from the floor and reappear on her hand. She slowly turns her hand palm up. Her little nose wrinkles, and she grins with glee as she finds she is holding a sunbeam in her hand. With a squeal of delight she races back and forth gathering the sunbeams one by one — a bouquet of sunshine!

The rewards of motherhood come in tiny surprise packages — packages of love like a bouquet of sunshine. And it seems they're always wrapped inside a gray day. Not necessarily a gray and cloudy day, but rather a foggy one on my heart. A day when the everyday drudgery of housewifery and motherhood suddenly hits me on the head.

An A-number-one-gray-day is when I think if I see one more dish with egg dried on it — I will scream! If I have to wipe up one more glass of spilt milk — I will cry! If I have to pick up one more toy (than the 10,000 I've already picked up) from in front of the bathroom door — I will tear out my hair!

It seems the Lord must know when these little surprise packages of love will be most appreciated because that's precisely when they appear. They slip up and tap me on the shoulder, just in time to chase the gloom from my heart. They are tiny packages that fill my heart with the joy of

a spontaneous hug and wet baby kiss with
    a soft whisper "I yuv oo, mommy!"
a tinkling jangle of piano keys and a happy
    little voice singing her own rendition of
"Jesus Loves Me" — slightly mixed into
    "Row, Row, Row Your Boat,"
a shared giggling joke — bringing gales of
    ringing laughter from us both,
a tiny voice saying a good-night prayer
    in the soft darkness of her room with
    a chirping, "Thank oo, God, for mommy."

Each little package is a separate blossom in a bouquet of sunshine, wrapped in love and tied with the satin ribbon of a gentle memory. And special enough to make me realize — motherhood has no greater reward than

itself.

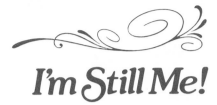

I'm Still Me!

I'm a wife.

I'm a mother.

But where is the-me-who-used-to-be?

The me who likes to sit barefoot in the sweet, warm grass in the backyard and think. Or not think if a nonthinking mood strikes. Not so much as a book or a cup of coffee in my hands — just me, the old oak tree, and maybe a bird or two.

The me who likes treetop watching, to raise my gaze from horizontal to vertical. To observe the artful delicacy of woven leaf patterns. To hunt for acorns or pinecones and other hidden treasures peeking down at me from above. To absorb strength from the straight towering trunk of a pine or the gnarled and scarred curvature of an oak.

The me who likes to communicate with birds — the little brown ones whose name, class, and status remain unknown to me, but they don't care and neither do I. It is enough to remain quiet and still and let them speak to me.

The me who finds joy in flowers — to lie flat on my stomach eyeball-to-eyeball with a sweet pea. To memorize its ruffled outline, its delicate thickness, its angle in the sun, its own inimitable variation in hue, its gentle twisting as it listens to the breeze.

The me who giggles inside at the sight of ivy pushing its way through a crack in a concrete wall. As though its obstinate will to live and grow far exceeds man's efforts to dominate. Hooray for ivy!

In the rush of recent months I've somehow forgotten about the-me-who-used-to-be. She's hiding somewhere behind a bucket of dirty diapers, or behind a book on child rearing, or sacked-out in the easy chair, totally exhausted. She needs to be awakened and given the precious gift of a tap on the shoulder and a gentle shove into her world that used to be.

It's still there

you know.

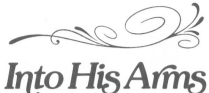

Into His Arms

Then he took the children into his arms and placed his hands on their heads and he blessed them.

Mark 10:16 (LB)

I like to close my eyes and imagine myself a child on the day Jesus blessed the little ones.

I can see the emerald water of the Sea of Galilee sparkling in the distance. Here and there a fish jumps, showing a silver-streaked side to the sun. I can feel the salty sea breeze against my sun-flushed face and hear the gulls calling to each other as they soar and glide on the wind.

There is a hot, dusty throng gathered on a grassy knoll with Jesus seated in the center. From the edge of the crowd I catch a glimple of His face, and something is written there that makes my heart want to soar like the birds overhead. I long to come closer, but the crowd is gathered tightly around Him, listening so intently that they pay little attention to the child in their midst. I begin weaving my way toward Him through the maze of long-robed giants.

Finally there is a clearing. Jesus turns and looks at me with happy eyes. And the clear, tender love I see there quickens my heart — I rush to Him, feeling my heart will burst if I lose a moment.

Suddenly there are huge men standing in front of me, blocking my way. They tell me not to bother Jesus, that He is much too busy to take time for me! My little heart heavy with disappointment, I turn to trudge away.

Then I hear a voice — gentler than a lamb's and stronger than a lion's — telling them to let me come to Him. And I feel His big strong arms around me as He lifts me up and holds me close. I nestle in His lap with my cheek resting against the soft homespun folds of His robe. I can feel the warmth of His arms around me as He softly kisses the top of my sun-warmed head.

> *Jesus — not just a name, but a person.*
> *A person so real I can reach out and touch Him*
> *and climb up into His lap.*
> *Jesus — not just a name, but the source of love.*
> *He was love by Galilee,*
> *He was love at Calvary,*
> *He is love today.*
> *He is love waiting. Waiting to hear the whisper of*
> *a child crying out to Him.*
> *Waiting to hold me close to His*
> *heart if I but whisper His name —*
> *Jesus!*

His love for my child is the same as it was for those He blessed on that day so long ago. Someday she can hold outstretched arms to Him,
whisper His name,
and be cuddled in His everlasting
arms of love.

Security Is Knowing Love Is Forever

A man had two sons. When the younger told his father, "I want my share of your estate now, instead of waiting until you die!" his father agreed to divide his wealth between his sons.

A few days later this younger son packed all his belongings and took a trip to a distant land, and there wasted all his money on parties and prostitutes. About the time his money was gone a great famine swept over the land, and he began to starve. He persuaded a local farmer to hire him to feed his pigs. The boy became so hungry that even the pods he was feeding the swine looked good to him. And no one gave him anything.

When he finally came to his senses, he said to himself, "At home even the hired men have food enough and to spare, and here I am, dying of hunger! I will go home to my father and say, 'Father, I have sinned against both heaven and you, and am no longer worthy of being called your son. Please take me on as a hired man.'"

So he returned home to his father. And while he was still a long distance away, his father saw him coming, and was filled with loving pity and ran and embraced him and kissed him.

His son said to him. "Father, I have sinned against heaven and you, and am not worthy of being called your son —"

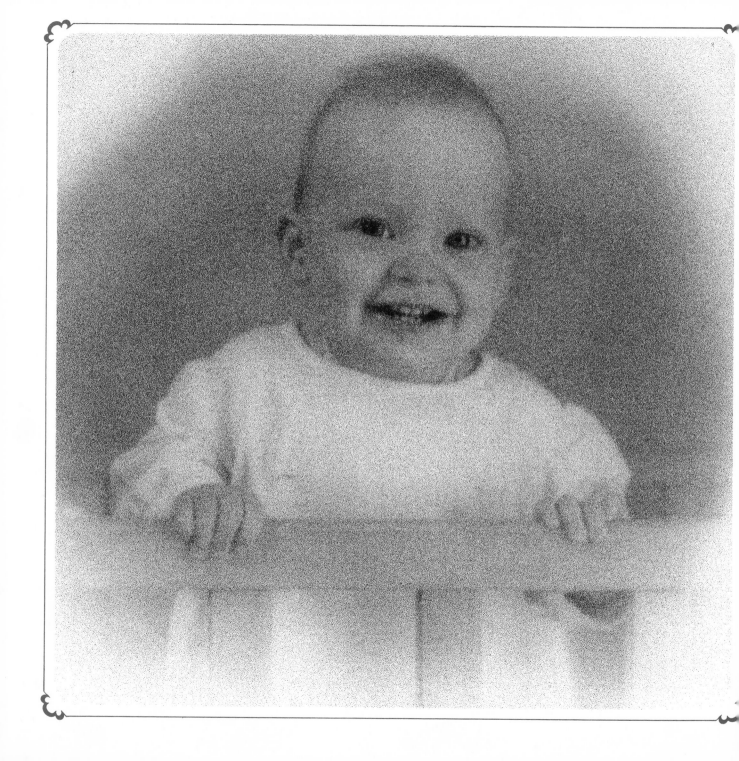

But his father said to the slaves, "Quick! Bring the finest robe in the house and put it on him. And a jeweled ring for his finger; and shoes! And kill the calf we have in the fattening pen. We must celebrate with a feast, for this son of mine was dead and has returned to life. He was lost and is found."

Luke 15:11-24 (LB)

My little girl stoops by her dolly cradle, patting a well-worn and smudged Raggedy Ann while she sings something vaguely reminiscent of "Rock-a-bye Baby." Love swells within my heart as I watch her play. My love for her is so deep and strong I can't imagine not loving her forever.

I think about unconditional love, the kind of love portrayed in the story of the prodigal son. What if my little girl, like the prodigal son, decides in future years to sprout her wings and fly into sin and immorality? Will my love be so deep that I would never stop loving her — or even *threaten* to stop loving her — no matter what? And would I welcome her back with arms full of love and forgiveness?

Somehow, just thinking about it makes me feel terribly vulnerable.

Then the thought occurs to me that *I* am loved with an unconditional love! Regardless of my mistakes, weaknesses, or failures, God is standing with arms outstretched — just waiting for me to turn around and run to Him. He will wrap me in His coat of forgiveness and place the jeweled ring of His unending love upon my finger.

What a magnificent pattern for unconditional love! If my heavenly Father can love *me* with a love like that, can I not follow in His footsteps and, in turn, love my daughter with the same unchanging, unconditional love? A love and acceptance that will permeate her innermost being with no strings attached?

As my little girl grows in the knowledge that she is loved no matter what, she will also be learning what it is like to be loved unconditionally by her heavenly Father. And her greatest security will be in the knowledge that

His love is forever.

Making Memories

I remember waking one dark and scary night when I was a tiny child. A terrifying nightmare had crept into my childish dreams, and I cried out into the spooky silence of the night. I'll never forget feeling the comforting arms of my father surround me as he lifted me from my bed to sit on his lap. He held me close and prayed the Lord's Prayer with me, and I fell asleep against his big, strong shoulder, all traces of fear erased.

Memories —
  beautiful and loving memories to cherish.

My child will have memories, too. And in these early years of her life her daddy and mommy are her memories. Every day of her life she gives us a blank piece of canvas on which we paint thoughts, dreams, and experiences — all separate brush strokes in the painting of a memory.

I stand now at the window and watch my little daughter toddle down the walk with her daddy. Even the bright sunlight playing on the red and golden leaves of autumn cannot match the shining pride illuminating her pixie face. Joyful expectation and a huge sense of importance emanate from her tiny figure as she reaches up to take daddy's hand. I watch as they stoop beside a little brown bird happily splashing in a puddle of water.

Memories —

I can see them now across the street at the park. I suppress a giggle as daddy zooms down the slide with a little blond bundle on his lap. I can hear her squeals of glee from here. I watch the wind catch her hair as daddy swings her higher and higher. Her cheeks turn bright and rosy as she races back and forth from sandbox to merry-go-round. The joy of her excitement is catching. Her daddy tosses her in the air amid more squeals of delight, then holds her close as he carries her home.

Memories —

It's twilight now, and the crisp autumn air has brought with it the occasion of lighting the fireplace for the first time this season. Our little family sits on the warm, soft carpet in front of the hearth, eating popcorn and crisp red apples. Just a special time before bedtime for our little girl. A special time of stories and songs (punctuated with little chirps of "no-bed-yet!").

Memories —

How much will this child remember of her early years? I know she is too young to remember much of anything, but perhaps these experiences are the first sketches for the paintings her memory will hold years from now.

Beautiful and loving memories to cherish.

A Lamb for My Angel

he twinkling lights on the fragrant pine towering in the corner of the living room match the glistening in my eyes, and the fragrance of the season seems to overwhelm me with feelings of love, excitement, and a touch of nostalgia — feelings that nearly always bring quick, warm tears to my eyes.

It's late. The house is quiet with sleepiness. I turn out the lights, leaving only the Christmas tree standing aglow, winking at the flickering embers in the fireplace. I curl up on the rug in front of the fire, toasting my toes with its warmth. I don't want these tender and peaceful moments on a late Christmas Eve to escape. My thoughts drift dreamily —

Just a moment ago I tiptoed quietly into the nursery to peek at my little angel sleeping soundly in her crib. Sprawled out flat on her back with arms outstretched, she reminded me of "angels" I made as a child by flopping backwards into a snowbank and moving my arms up and down — making wings on the image left in the snow.

It's hard to believe tomorrow will be her third Christmas. I remember the awe and wonder of her first Christmas just two short years ago. What a Christmas gift she was at five weeks old. A little package of love from heaven!

And I think of that magnificent gift God gave to all of us nearly two thousand years ago. The babe born in a stable, sent to redeem us.

In my human reasoning, I try to imagine the depth and spectrum of God's love brought into focus in the form of baby Jesus. As a human parent I know how deeply I care for this child of mine, so I try to comprehend the multiplied and *perfect* love the Father had for His infant Son born in Bethlehem that night so long ago.

My thoughts drift to the plans and dreams I have for my little girl. I think about the choices she will have to make in the future. A mother has the right and privilege to *dream* about the wonderful opportunities that may be afforded her child, but her child has the right to *choose* which paths to take. So as I sit here cozily in front of the fire, I think about the bright hope she has for tomorrow.

Once again my thoughts bounce back to that baby in the manger. Jesus. I wonder if Mary knew what would happen to her Son during His lifetime on earth. She knew that He was God's Son on a magnificent mission — to save us all from our sins. But did she know *how* He would do this? Did she know He would suffer? And die so utterly alone on that cross?

But God knew. All of His love had been poured out into the form of that baby lying in the hay among the cattle and sheep that night. Oh, the compassion and tenderness He must have felt as He gazed down upon His little Son. And as the panorama of Jesus' life flashed in front of Him, what terrible anguish He must have felt as He knew what was already planned for that babe lying so peacefully asleep.

How much God must love me! To allow His beloved Son, Jesus Christ, to suffer and die a tortuous death on the cross for *me* — for everyone — all the generations of the world that have been and are yet to come.

The gray-orange embers are slowly dying. Just a soft glow remains as I turn out the Christmas lights and tiptoe down the hall. I stop at the nursery door to make one last check before going to bed.

As I gaze in at the little form clutching her fuzzy "Lambie-pie" close to her face, I think again of God's sacrifice. I picture Jesus dying on the cross. What if I

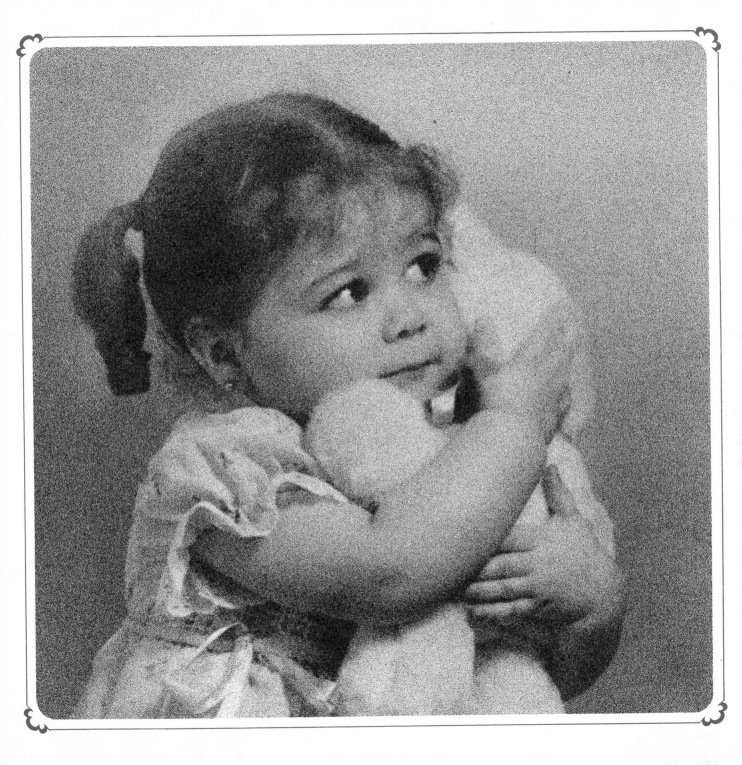

had to sacrifice my daughter? I can't even imagine the love, the *perfect* love that would take. But another thought quickly jumps into my mind — it is not necessary. Jesus paid it all. He is the sacrificed Lamb. Another lamb will never be necessary.

His death on the cross did not conquer Him. He conquered death once and for all when that giant stone was rolled away from His tomb and He was gloriously resurrected.

Resurrected!

Never again will God's creation be subjected to the threat of death. By believing in Jesus Christ and His atonement for our sins, we can be saved from death and have eternal life.

I stoop over the crib and plant a soft kiss upon that tousled head. Again I think of her future — her bright future. For I love her, but my love for her doesn't begin to compare with God's beautiful and tender love for her.

And that is the greatest gift she will ever receive: God's love in the form of that precious Lamb — Jesus.

A Season Passes

I sit propped against the trunk of our old, gnarled oak in the backyard. The soft glow of the fading sun reflects on the shimmering umbrella of leaves above my head.

At my side is a little girl, her babyhood fading as quickly as the setting sun. The fingers of the dying rays tie glowing ribbons in her hair. Her upturned face, rosy in its fresh and innocent youthfulness, solemnly gazes at the colorful glory of the gold and purple sunset.

I take her chubby, tanned hand in mine. It seems only yesterday that this childish hand was the tightly clenched fist of a newborn infant. How quickly the season of infancy has passed. My baby is a child now.

Time has an almost magical quality of standing still and then slipping up behind you. With each baby stage I think time has been captured and she will never change — that she will remain forever the way she is this moment. Then time subtly taps me on the shoulder, and my clouded eyes open to the beautiful transformation of my little rosebud.

She is changing and growing and becoming. Time does not stop for her. Like a tiny computer, she is being programed each moment of every day for what she will be the rest of her life. Bit by bit her daddy and I are filling her heart and soul with pieces of ourselves. And these pieces are being stored away in the depth of

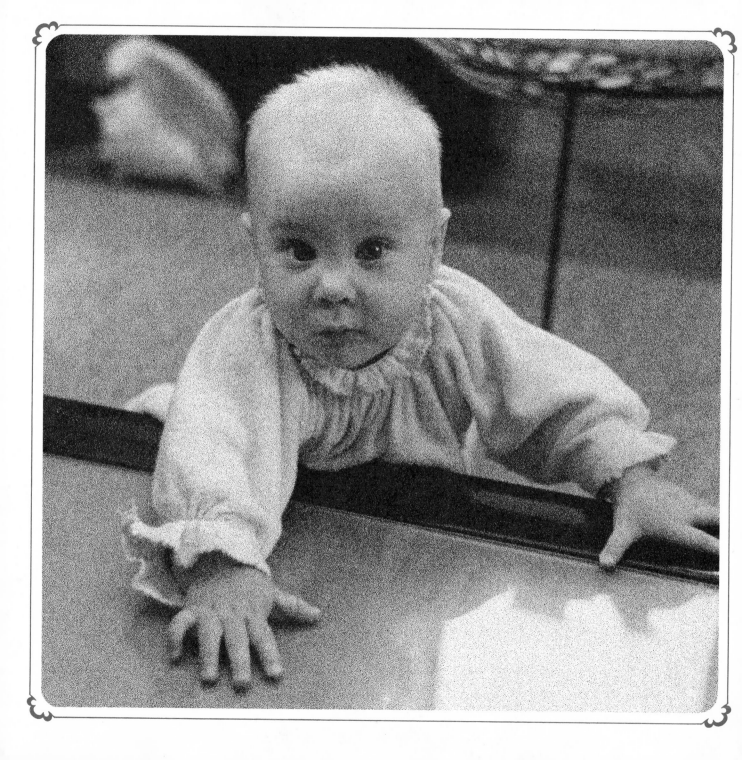

her little being. Not simply as memories (although these remain, too), but something infinitely more important. That which we are —

honest . . . or dishonest
patient . . . or impatient
kind . . . or unkind
responsible . . . or irresponsible
believing . . . or unbelieving
loving . . .or unloving —
our child is becoming.

By wiggling skills through her fingers and toes
into herself,
By picking up habits and attitudes of those
around her,
By pushing and pulling her own world —
Thus a child learns.

Through trial
more through trial than error,
more through pleasure than pain,
more through experience than suggestion,
more through suggestion than direction —
Thus a child learns.

Through affection
through love
through patience
through understanding
through belonging
through doing
through being —
Thus a child learns.

Day by day the child comes
to know a little bit of what you know,
to think a little bit of what you think,
to understand your understanding.
That which you dream
and believe
and are
In truth — becomes the child.

The fading sun slips from the lavender sky pulling down the shade of twilight with its pale stars and watery moon. I hold a precious wee hand to my cheek and kiss the smudges of dirt on its soft baby palm.

How much can this small hand hold?
Not much really.
But her heart?
It can hold all of ourselves
and more.